MW01293972

The 14-Day Sugar Detox Diet

Step-By-Step Meal Plan And Recipes To Kick Sugar Cravings, Lose Weight Easily, And Feel Amazing!

Sarah Givens

DISCLAIMER
The information presented on this site is provided for informational purposes only, it is not meant to substitute for medical advice or diagnosis provided by your physician or other medical professional. Do not use this information to diagnose, treat or cure any illness or health condition. If you have, or suspect that you have a medical problem, contact your physician or health care provider.

The author and/or any of their proprietors assume no liability for any injury, illness or adverse affects caused by the misuse and/or use of the information or products presented in this book.

DEDICATION

To Kevin for being the first person to help me understand that we have way more control over our health than we are led to believe.

CONTENTS

Introduction   i

Chapter I   Falling Under Sugar's Spell   1

Chapter II   The Not-So-Sweet Facts   5

Chapter III   The Sweetness Scam   11

Chapter IV   Breaking the Sugar Cycle   15

Chapter V   Back In Control in 21 Days   21

Chapter VI   Low-Sugar Living   27

                 Mayo   28

                 Tartar Sauce   28

                 Salad Dressings   29

                 Cauliflower Rice   30

                 Faux Tortillas   31

                 Veggie Noodles   32

                 Gussied-Up Greek Yogurt   33

                 Chicken Mushroom Salad   34

                 Roasted Shrimp with Garlic   35

                 3-Bite Frittatas   36

                 Roasted Asparagus Soup   37

                 Pulled Garlic Pork w/ Cauli-Rice   38

Protein Shake · 39

Bulletproof Coffee® · 40

Chicken w/ Artichokes & Olives · 41

Simple Chicken Soup · 42

Poached Fish · 43

Roasted Veggies · 44

Avocado Egg Salad · 45

Spaghetti Squash & Meatballs · 46

Scotch Eggs · 47

Chicken Salad · 48

Spring Rolls with Nut Sauce · 49

    Nut Sauce · 49

Stuffed Steak · 51

3-Bean Chili [slow cooker] · 52

Apple & Olive Spinach Salad · 53

Green Chili Salmon Muffins · 54

Moroccan Chicken with Lemon · 55

Ham-arrito · 56

Cauli Tabbouleh · 57

Wasabi Crab Cakes · 58

Wasabi Sauce 58

Tuna Salad 59

Chicken Quick Stir Fry 60

Sausage Breakfast Casserole 61

Waldorf Chicken Salad 62

Devilled Eggs 62

Sausage Red Curry Stroganoff 63

Mushroom-Broccoli Soup 64

Seafood Balls 65

Baked Oatmeal 67

Orange-Berry Salad 68

Tomatillo Pulled Pork [slow cooker] 69

Chili Con Carne 70

Cobb Salad 71

Squash Soup [slow cooker] 72

Antipasto Kabobs 73

Oat Cakes 74

Sweet Success! 75

Sarah Givens

INTRODUCTION

Have you noticed lately how everyone is talking about sugar like it's a dangerous drug? Please say it isn't so. Sugar is our favorite comfort food. It's how we celebrate holidays, outings, and special occasions. It's how we end our meals and begin our romances. It's our ice cream, box of chocolates, birthday cake, and funnel cake at the fair. How can something that delightful be bad for us?

But quite honestly, those things aren't really the major problem for most people. When we gobble down a banana split, we already know that we've eaten a lot of sugar, right? It's a 'treat' and not an everyday thing.

The real problem is the quantity of sugar we consume without being aware of it. The amount of sugar that's 'hidden' under various names in our everyday life, even things like toothpaste, is astonishing… and frightening.

Too much of anything is usually bad news, and sugar is no exception. Overexposure has the effect of desensitizing you. Your tolerance level is raised. It becomes a vicious circle. The more sugar you consume, the less you experience the sweetness of it… so you need to increase the amount of sugar to get the same sweet taste. You constantly need more sugar to get the same effect. Hmm, that sounds eerily like what happens with drug addicts, doesn't it?

Whether sugar is actually 'addictive' is a hotly debated topic right now, but one thing is not in question. As our consumption of sugar has risen, our level of health has declined. For decades, fats have been called the 'bad guys' --- blamed for making us overweight and causing heart disease along with host of other health problems. Recent scientific research, however, is showing that fats have been falsely accused. The real culprit is most likely sugar.

What can you do about it? That's what you'll learn in this

book. You'll learn how sugar negatively affects your mind and body, and why artificial sweeteners are even worse for you. You'll learn the many names that these substances hide behind, and how to find and avoid them. Most importantly, you'll learn how to break free from excessive sugar consumption, how to 'detox', and then how to reset your sweetness sensors back to natural and normal levels.

Finally, you'll learn how to maintain a lower-sugar lifestyle so you can continue to enjoy clearer skin, better sleep, less body fat, better digestion, better overall health, fewer headaches and body aches, longer life. Yes, you can have your cake and eat it too. All you need to do now is just turn the page!

CHAPTER I: FALLING UNDER SUGAR'S SPELL

That sugar has cast a spell over humankind cannot be denied. Since it was first domesticated over 10,000 years ago, sugar has been credited with mystical powers, touted as a medical remedy, been a status symbol, and slowly spread its sticky tentacles all over the globe. Man had evolved to be a superior processor of fructose, once only available in seasonal fruit, and our bodies were designed to crave it and to store it as fat, to protect us from starving in the winter. Sugar made that substance available year round, feeding our instinctive cravings and, as it became both more available and more affordable, we became infatuated with sugar.

The first to fall for sugar were the New Guinea tribesmen, who discovered that chewing a stem of sugar cane produced a totally new and enticing burst of flavor. They cultivated the plants, and sugar became an integral part of their ancient myths and featured heavily in their religious ceremonies. Knowledge of this wondrous plant slowly spread from one island to another.

Sugar cane arrived on the mainland of Asia around 1000 B.C., and from there, the magic of sugar continued to spread westward. In India, sugar cane was refined into the form we know today, sugar. How to make sugar from sugar cane was a secret process, passed carefully from masters to apprentices, but by 600 A.D. the rulers of the Persian Empire were dazzling their guests with all sorts of sugared treats. The conquering Arab armies were themselves enthralled by sugar, and they took both the plants and the knowledge of how to refine sugar home with them. "Wherever they went, the Arabs brought with them sugar, the product and the technology of its production," wrote Sidney Mintz in Sweetness and Power (Viking Press, 1985).

The Arabs also turned sugar production from a secret art into an industry. The work was so physically difficult that slaves and prisoners of war made up the bulk of the workforce. The European Crusaders who returned home brought with them memories of sugar, and European noblemen began to trade with the Muslim caliphs for sugar since it couldn't be grown in Europe. The amount available was very small, and sugar was considered a luxury spice. As the Ottoman Empire spread in the 1400's, trade with the Mid-East became much more difficult, and sugar was very scarce in Europe.

However, the European elite had fallen under sugar's spell and they were not about to give it up easily. The many European explorers of the 15th century were looking for other sources for spices, with sugar ranking high on that list. The Portuguese took sugar cane to the Atlantic islands that they colonized and Columbus planted the first sugar cane in the New World on his second voyage. The rain forests of this New World were ideally suited for growing cane. Sugar was about to 'boom'.

The Caribbean Islands, and later Brazil, became centers of sugar production, and this increased production had two terrible results. The first was that the price of sugar fell, since there was much more of it available, and because it was more affordable, the demand for it rose. Sugar was no longer a luxury but became a household staple, not only for the nobility but also for the growing middle-class. By the mid-

1600's, even the poor would have access to sugar, and it began to be eaten much more often with long-term effects on health. As early as 1675, the British physician Thomas Willis noted a rise in diabetes in England.

The other result was that the sugar plantations needed a lot of workers, and the European nations did not have prisoners-of-war to meet the demand. Sugar became one side of the Triangular Trade: sugar to Europe in exchange for manufactured goods, manufactured goods to Africa for slaves, slaves to the Americas to work the cane fields and sugar pressing sheds. Over half of the African slaves brought to the Americas worked on the sugar plantations. In fact, sugar was one of the first products to be boycotted by those opposed to slavery. The early Quaker abolitionists refused to sell or use slave-produced sugar, and they actively urged others to do the same.

Unfortunately, the sugar train was rolling and there was no stopping it. Even sugar cane couldn't give us enough sugar, so we found a way to get it from sugar beets as well! The British common man ate 4 pounds of sugar a year in 1700. That amount increased to 18 pounds a year on average by 1800. By 1870, it was up to 47 pounds, and by 1900, 100 pounds annually --- more than doubling in just 30 years! Today, for all our 'health consciousness', sources say the average American still consumes at least 77 pounds of sugar each year, with some estimates going as high as 165 pounds. That's added sugar, by the way, not the sugar that occurs naturally in other foods we eat like fruit.

The insidious thing about sugar is that the more you eat, the more you want... and need. That craving for more sweets caused by sugar is one of the reasons behind the current hot debate over whether it's actually addictive. Sugar has been compared to cocaine and heroine, and one well-publicized scientific study has indicated that sugar is four times as addictive as those two drugs. Sugar stimulates the same part of the brain as those two drugs, and in the same way. If you normally consume a lot of sugar and stop 'cold turkey', you're likely to experience physical withdrawal symptoms. It's also perfectly legal and hidden in an alarming amount of what you eat every day. The food industry continues to add more and more sugar to foods, under a thousand aliases, precisely *because* it keeps you coming back for more.

Like the evil queen in a fairy story, sugar has ensnared and enchanted us as she has spread her influence around the world. Men have traded for her, explored for her, enslaved for her, and killed for her. We find it hard to resist her siren's call, despite growing evidence that she's killing us. It's time to break free and take back control of your food and your health. It's time to detox and end the sweet misery that sugar has wrought.

CHAPTER II: THE NOT-SO-SWEET FACTS

The sugar you know is actually a complex sugar called sucrose, and it's composed of 12 atoms of carbon, 22 atoms of hydrogen, and 11 atoms of oxygen ($C_{12}H_{22}O_{11}$). It's a carbohydrate, as are all foods containing those three elements, and it's found naturally in most plants. Sugarcane and sugar beets are particularly rich in sucrose, and their juice is processed into crystalline sugar. Sucrose breaks down into two simpler sugars: fructose and glucose. There's actually a ring of each one in sucrose, joined by oxygen, so they are easily separated. Fructose is the type of sugar found in fruit; glucose is your body's fuel of choice for energy.

For most of human history, summer was 'feast' and winter was 'famine'. Our systems needed to store fat to see us through the winter. We therefore developed a great survival ability to store fructose from summer's bounty as fat, and to later use that stored energy to supplement winter's meager food supply. It worked great until the growth of agriculture, when we no longer had to rely so much on stored fat for survival. However, biologically, we continue to be great at storing fructose and burning glucose.

When sugar (sucrose) entered the picture, its structure provided for both functions. Sucrose gives us glucose for energy and fructose to make fat... but in the modern world, we don't need the stored fat anymore. Beginning in the mid-1800's, our sugar intake increased dramatically, giving us far more fructose than nature ever intended, and our sugar consumption has continued to rise steadily. Being overweight began to become an issue in developed countries.

In the 1930's, Dr. Haven Emerson of Columbia University noted the link between the increased sugar consumption between 1900 and 1920 and the corresponding number of deaths from diabetes. In the 1960's, John Yudkin, a British nutrition expert, found a link between high sugar intake and high levels of fat and insulin in the blood, known risk factors for heart disease as well as diabetes. His study, however, sank beneath those of other scientists who were blaming dietary fat, especially saturated fats, for the alarming rise in obesity and heart disease. The low-fat movement had begun.

Since the 1970's we eat far less fat than before, yet the percentage of the population suffering from high blood pressure, heart disease, diabetes, and obesity has continued to grow. According to Richard Johnson of the University of Colorado-Denver, in 1980 there were 153 million people that had diabetes. By 2013 that number had climbed to 347 million."Why is it that one-third of adults [worldwide] have high blood pressure, when in 1900 only 5percent had high blood pressure?" Johnson asks... "Sugar, we believe, is one of the culprits, if not the major culprit." (Cohen, Rich. "Sugar Love". *National Geographic Magazine*. August 2013.) Sugar has also been implicated in dementia, Alzheimer's, and macular degeneration.

There are numerous scientific studies underway looking at the link between sugar and serious health problems. More and more researchers and medical professionals are coming to share Yudkin's view that fat is not the bad boy, sugar is, and more and more people are turning to low-carb diets to reclaim their health.

Short-Term Effects of Sugar

Empty Calories

Sugar is pure energy, and that means calories. Unlike other foods, however, sugar carries no essential nutrients whatsoever. No proteins, minerals, vitamins, amino acids, or fat --- just calories, which is why they are called 'empty' calories. So consuming sugar gives you lots of calories without any physical benefit; it provides nothing for your body to use to repair itself or fight off disease. It stimulates the pleasure centers in your brain and encourages you to eat more of it, but it gives back nothing except tooth decay. The bad bacteria in your mouth gobble it up and thrive, although you may be heading for nutritional deficiencies. If more than about 10% of your calories are coming from sugar, this can seriously impact your health and your weight.

Elevated Triglycerides

Remember that sugar (sucrose) breaks down into glucose and fructose? We don't actually need very much fructose. The liver metabolizes it, and if needed, it's turned into glycogen and stored. Most people already have enough glycogen, however, so the liver converts that fructose into fats called triglycerides, a major risk factor for heart disease. When your liver has as much of these fats as it can hold (fatty liver is a health problem of its own), the triglycerides are leaked out into your blood stream. If you've had a cholesterol test done, it measures not only HDL and LDL but also triglycerides. Lots of people have elevated levels of triglycerides, and it's because of sugar, not dietary fat.

Hunger

Fructose has yet another bad effect on us --- it doesn't satisfy. In a study done at the Yale University School of Medicine and published in the *Journal of the American Medical Association* in 2013, it was found that fructose doesn't promote a feeling of fullness like glucose does. Another study showed that fructose doesn't lower the hormone ghrelin, which stimulates hunger. The end result is that consuming fructose doesn't satisfy your hunger, so you'll eat more.

Insulin Resistance

Glucose, the other half of sugar, causes the release of insulin, which controls the glucose levels in the blood. Continual high levels of insulin cause the cells of the body to become resistant to its effect, overdosed if you will. This forces your system to release even more insulin to achieve the necessary effect. Insulin resistance is believed to be the precursor for quite a large number of diseases such as metabolic syndrome, cardiovascular disease, and of course Type 2 diabetes. Consuming too much glucose is what sets this process in motion.

Addiction

Sugar causes a huge release of dopamine in the brain, much more than happens with other foods found in nature. Dopamine is a neurotransmitter that controls our reward and pleasure centers. It also helps to regulate emotional responses and produces that 'pride in achievement' feeling. Falling in love causes a big release of dopamine and, for a lot of people, so does riding roller coasters and participating in risky activities like bungee jumping or skydiving. But dopamine is a 'high' and not meant to be a normal state for your body. People can easily become addicted to that high, whether it comes from cocaine or sugar, particularly if they are naturally low on dopamine to begin with. Scientific studies are ongoing, but current indications are that sugar is more addictive than cocaine.

Long-Term Effects

Obesity

The increased consumption of empty calories from sugar, combined with a less physically demanding lifestyle to burn off those calories, has resulted in the alarming rise of obesity. The effect of sugar on hormones such as insulin, dopamine, ghrelin, and others, almost programs your system to gain weight, and it also keeps you from losing it. Many are blaming carbohydrates in general for this phenomenon, but many studies have shown a strong link between sugar and obesity, especially in children. A study conducted by Dr. David S Ludwig of Children's Hospital in Boston, MA, indicated a 60% increased risk of obesity in children for every serving of sugar-sweetened beverage consumed daily. Other studies have shown similar results across all age groups.

Heart Disease

More and more scientific studies are showing that eating fats is not responsible for the rise in heart disease. The finger is now pointing directly at sugar. Food manufacturers have lowered the fat content of their products and, to maintain taste, they've replaced it with various forms of sugar, like high-fructose corn syrup [HFCS]. In the past 30 years, this has greatly increased the amount of sugar, especially fructose, which we consume. Fructose, as you remember, produces triglycerides. As we've eaten less fat and more sugar, the rate of heart disease has continued to climb, and it is now the # 1 killer worldwide.

Studies have also linked sugar with high blood pressure, elevated cholesterol levels, and other risk factors for cardiovascular disease. It appears that sugar, particularly in the form of fructose, has a horrible effect on metabolism, and it is quite possibly the major contributor to the rise in heart disease.

Type II Diabetes

The resistance of cells to the effects of insulin forces the pancreas to produce more and more of it in an attempt to control high blood sugar, which has its own dangers. Raised insulin levels can produce more insulin resistance. It's a vicious cycle and eventually the pancreas just can't keep up. Blood sugar reaches dangerous levels, and Type 2 diabetes is diagnosed. Type 2 diabetes raises the risk of stroke, heart disease, and kidney failure, and is the #7 cause of death. Its non-fatal effects include obesity, blindness, cognitive degeneration, and poor blood circulation that often results in the need for amputations.

Metabolic Syndrome

Metabolic Syndrome, also known as Syndrome X, is a group of symptoms that, taken together, indicate a *very* high risk for developing cardiovascular diseases and/or diabetes. Identified less than 20 years ago, it is estimated that one in every four people may have metabolic syndrome ('Are You at Risk for Metabolic Syndrome?' WebMD, 2013). Abdominal fat, high blood sugar, high blood pressure, and unhealthy cholesterol levels are the factors in diagnosing metabolic syndrome. It doubles your risk of cardiovascular disease, and it increases your risk for developing diabetes by five times. Most of those symptoms are related to sugar consumption.

Cancer

Cancer is the #2 cause of death around the world, and sugar appears to play a starring role. Although the exact causes of various cancers are still being studied, two potential factors are insulin levels and inflammation. Both are strongly affected by sugar consumption through its effect on metabolism and hormones. Several studies have shown that having high insulin levels greatly increases the risk of developing cancer, and the metabolism of fructose is known to increase inflammation throughout the system.

As you've seen, the effects of sugar on your health are really not sweet at all. We're all familiar with the energy crash that follows the sugar high, making us too tired for physical activity, but that's just the beginning. The American Heart Association now warns us to reduce consumption because sugar is 'empty' calories, which doesn't go nearly far enough in the opinion of many researchers. "It has nothing to do with its calories," says endocrinologist Robert Lustig of the University of California, San Francisco. "Sugar is a poison by itself when consumed at high doses." (Cohen, Rich. "Sugar Love".*National Geographic Magazine*. August 2013.)

CHAPTER III: THE SWEETNESS SCAM

So, are artificial sweeteners the answer? Unfortunately, not! In fact, they appear to be even more hazardous than actual sugar. The first no-calorie artificial sweetener, saccharin, was discovered in 1878 by a chemist (working with coal tar, a known carcinogen --- eew!). Public health officials of that time questioned its safety, and we still don't have a definitive answer to that question. Studies funded by the manufacturers showed that artificial sweeteners are not harmful in any way; studies funded by the sugar industry show all sorts of problems. The facts, long buried under these conflicting claims, are finally starting to surface ... and they're not pretty.

Artificial sweeteners appear to be a health hazard, disguised as a benefit and foisted upon the public. The only promise they live up to is that they add no calories. There are five chemically produced artificial sweeteners that have been approved for use in food: saccharin [Sweet 'N Low]; aspartame [Equal, NutraSweet]; sucralose [Splenda]; acesulfame potassium (Ace K) [Sweet One, Sunett]; and neotame. They are found, not only in diet sodas, but also in everything from 'light' apple juice to yogurt. Many products contain both sugar and artificial sweeteners!

The main problem with non-caloric artificial sweeteners

(NAS) is that you can't fool your metabolism --- you can only mess it up. Whether or not NAS are carcinogenic, and that debate is still raging in the medical and scientific communities, these substances don't help anyone lose weight. Really! Other health risks in using NAS cancel out the no calorie advantage. Let's look at those risks.

First, artificial sweeteners trick your system in several different ways. They are much sweeter than sugar or anything else found naturally in our food supply. Sucralose is 600 times sweeter than sugar, and neotame is 7000 times sweeter. Yes, you use much less of them to replace sugar, but their very intenseness dulls your taste buds. Natural sweetness somehow just doesn't taste as sweet anymore, and users are far more likely to consume more and sweeter foods.

The second trick is that when your taste buds signal 'sweet', your gut expects high calorie food to be coming its way. Your digestion prepares to deal with a lot of calories --- but it doesn't get them. All the wrong digestive hormones are waiting for that 'sweet' food, and consequently your digestion doesn't deal with the food efficiently. This is what causes many people to experience bloating, gas, and diarrhea when they consume artificial sweeteners, although folks often blame the food and not the NAS in it.

Recent research has also shown that NAS upset the balance of bacteria in the gut, killing off the good ones and allowing the more harmful to proliferate. Your gut is at the heart of your immune system, and throwing it out of whack is really not a good idea! The recent surge in ads for probiotics to 'reset' your gut shows just how many people have upset their digestive balance, most probably through consuming artificial sweeteners hidden in food. All the probiotics in the world can't help if they're killed off by NAS!

That 'sweet' signal sent by your taste buds also alerts your body to release insulin to control blood sugar levels. Since there's no sugar, only fake 'sweet', the insulin has nothing to do. It remains circulating until it has some sugar to deal with. This raises your risk of developing insulin resistance and diabetes, and it also increases your craving for sweets. It raises your production of ghrelin as well, causing you to feel hungrier.

Artificial sweeteners have also been found to contribute to weight gain in a number of studies. Recent research at the University of Texas found that diet soda drinkers were much more likely to become overweight than people who drank regular soda and they were 65% more likely to gain excess weight than those who didn't drink soda at all. This link between artificial sweeteners and weight gain has become so confirmed that the consumer advocate group US Right To Know has petitioned the government to prohibit the use of the word 'diet' with anything containing NAS. Gary Rushkin, the executive director of the group has said, "We have asked the FTC and FDA to shut down what appears to be a consumer fraud. We're hopeful they will stand with consumers and do the right thing." (Dr. Mercola, "Could This Headache Causing Neurotoxin Be on Its Way Out?'. Mercola.com, May 14, 2015.)

Most so-called 'natural' sweeteners suffer from many limitations as well. Many, such as agave nectar, are very high in fructose, and I've already discussed the problems with fructose. Sugar alcohols (sorbitol, xylitol, and mannitol) are being touted as an alternative, but like NAS they tend to cause a lot of digestive upset. Plant sugars, such as monk fruit and stevia, are often highly processed to make them crystalline like sugar, and that processing removes from them any pretense of being 'natural', no matter what the ads and packaging might say.

Raw honey was the sweetener commonly used before the sugar boom, and it's still a viable alternative. Unprocessed stevia is also good, but it can be hard to find except in liquid form. Read labels carefully.

Most sugar substitutes have been a scam, doing far more harm than good. They've tricked us into thinking we were eating healthier, and they've tricked our bodies into potentially lethal reactions. The evidence against them is mounting day by day. The catchphrase from the old TV ad for Chiffon margarine is certainly very true when it comes to artificial sweeteners --- 'It's not nice to fool Mother Nature!"

CHAPTER IV: BREAKING THE SUGAR CYCLE

The two previous chapters should have led you to understand why it's imperative that you break up with the Sugar Queen right now. While we've been blaming fat for our problems and avoiding its yummy richness, sugar has been stealthily stealing away with our health. But, breaking up with Miss Sugar is easier said than done, as you may already know.

Know your exit plan

Now that you know the problems that sugar can bring you, both short and long term, you're ready to begin, but there are several things that you need to do before you start the sugar detox. The first is to decide where you're going. You need to look ahead and decide how you intend to eat once you've broken free from sugar. The sugar detox is not a permanent lifestyle, so where do you want to end up? If you don't know which road you're taking, you'll end up back eating the same way you always have ... and you'll end up with the same problems all over again. Sugar detox is challenging, so make some permanent dietary changes while you're at it.

A diet that's low in carbohydrates will help to keep you away from sugar and on the right track to optimal health and well being, but there are a number of options out there. Do some research to find the one that best suits both you and your lifestyle. Atkins, Warrior, South Beach, Paleo, Stillman, ketogenic, Primal, or Zone ... *where are you headed?* What and how often do you want to eat? These are individual questions that only you can answer, and you can certainly tailor your own plan based on these diet plans and others.

Apart from having an end goal in sight, you will also need to customize the meal plan so you can transition into your preferred eating protocol easily. For instance, if you are headed towards a Paleo plan, you won't want to add grains like oatmeal and corn back into your menu during the third week of the detox. They're not Paleo, so you'll need to sub them out for more Paleo-friendly foods like eggs or cheese. Other diet plans will have you limiting the eggs but eating more dairy products. So, do your homework, decide where you're going, and begin to learn the plan. It will make your transition much easier, and it will keep you from backsliding.

AKA Sugar
Another thing you need to do to prepare for sugar detox is to learn the various names that sugar is listed under on food ingredient labels so you can avoid it. That's not as easy as it sounds. Package labels list the ingredient that forms the largest weight first, the second heaviest ingredient second, and so on. Many packaged foods have sugar listed under three or four different names so it doesn't show up so high in the list.

Let me give you an example. I have a package of instant mashed potatoes in front of me that I grabbed at random out of the pantry. What would you expect for the ingredients? I use potatoes, milk, butter, and a little salt to make mashed potatoes. Here's the label: potatoes, partially hydrogenated oil, corn syrup solids, salt, maltodextrin, coconut oil, nonfat dry milk, *sugar*, whey powder... we'll stop there. Do you put sugar in your mashed potatoes? It's the 8th ingredient ... but wait, it's actually also the 3rd ingredient [corn syrup solids] and the 5th ingredient [maltodextrin] as well. Three kinds of sugar? In mashed potatoes? That's definitely NOT going back into my pantry or onto my dinner plate!

This is a great example of the way that so much sugar is sneaking into your diet, as well as an object lesson in reading labels. Take your reading glasses when you go to the grocery store! Here are the most commonly used names that food manufacturers use for sugar:

Barley malt	Beet sugar	Brown sugar	Buttered syrup	Cane juice crystals	Cane sugar
Caramel	Corn syrup	Corn syrup solids	Confectioner's sugar	Carob syrup	Castor sugar
Date sugar	Demerara sugar	Dextran	Dextrose	Diastatic malt	Diatase
Ethyl maltol	Fructose	Fruit juice	Fruit juice concentrate	Galactose	Glucose
Glucose solids	Golden sugar	Golden syrup	Grape sugar	High-fructose corn syrup	Honey
Icing sugar	Invert sugar	Lactose	Maltodextrin	Maltose	Malt syrup
Mannitol	Maple syrup	Molasses	Muscovado	Panocha	Raw sugar
Refiner's syrup	Rice syrup	Sorbitol	Sorghum syrup	Sucrose	Sugar
Treacle	Turbinado	Yellow sugar	Xylitol		

Scary, huh? If you eliminate the ones that actually use the word 'sugar' in some way, it gets easier. If it ends in '–ose' or '-tol', it's probably sugar. 'Syrup' is a tip-off that it's sugar, as is the word 'cane', and if it has 'dextr' in it anywhere, it's also likely to be sugar. That should help. Know thy enemy and all his aliases!

Also brush up on the names of the artificial sweeteners because they may be listed by chemical name (aspartame) or brand name (NutraSweet).

Be Prepared

Finally, you'll need to do some personal preparation. Look through the meal plan and recipes. There are ingredients that you probably don't have in your pantry, such as almond or coconut flour and coconut aminos/liquid aminos, that you'll want to pick up. Watch for a sale on fresh frozen vegetables and stock your freezer. You may even want to crank up your crockpot and pre-cook some chicken to save prep time later. Practice grating cauliflower into rice and freeze it, too. These things will not only make you physically ready to prepare meals, but they will also help to make you mentally and emotionally ready.

Cutting back on sugar before you begin the detox and go cold turkey can make the first week much easier for you. If you drink a lot of soda, especially diet or caffeinated, wean yourself off of it now. Taking some small steps in advance, such as skipping desserts or cutting out sweet snacks, will help to take you off sugar a little more slowly.

It's also important to plan when you're going to start the detox. You need to expect some withdrawal symptoms, sometimes called the 'low carb flu', and you'll need to be able to accommodate them into your schedule. They usually start the second day, so factor that in. How they'll affect your work depends upon your job. Some people like to start on a Friday so they have the weekend to adjust; others find that adjusting while they're busy working is easier. Make sure to plan around holidays and family celebrations as well. It's better to schedule wisely and wait a few weeks to begin rather than to undermine your chance for success!

Possible Bumps in the Road

Let's talk about the withdrawal symptoms --- just what can you expect? Individual reaction varies widely depending not only on the level of sugar you've been used to having, but also on your personal biochemistry. Most people experience a few of the symptoms, often not all at once but spread out over a week or so. Most are mild and pass quickly, and knowing what's going on does a lot to make them easier to deal with. You'll experience most of the same things transitioning to any low-carb eating plan because your body converts most complex carbs like flour or potatoes into sugar!

Cravings

Most people experience carb cravings when they begin to detox. You're not just cutting out sugar, you know, but also all the other carbohydrates that your metabolism can easily convert to sugar. That's why it's called 'low carb flu'. Your best defense against these cravings is to fight them with other nutrients ---water, protein, and especially fat. Really increase your fat intake with butter, full-fat dairy, and avocado. Also lock up the sweet snacks! Cravings for carbs, and sugar in particular, usually become very manageable by the 5th day, so hang in there!

Headache

Many people also report having headaches from sugar withdrawal, just as they do when they quit caffeine. They're usually more a bother than truly painful. A visitor on mentalhealthdaily.com summed it nicely: "I'm on week number one of having completely stopped eating sugar. I am currently experiencing daily headaches... so consistent that I am taking 2 pills of Advil every four-six hours. Last night, just to ensure that the headaches are being caused by sugar withdrawal, I purposely ate a half spoon of sugar and immediately my headache went away. I am staying the course and will endure these headaches, which are not severe, just annoying." (Flores, Manuel. 11/23/2014. comments at http://mentalhealthdaily.com/2014/07/19/sugar-withdrawal-symptoms-list-of-possibilities/)

Irritability, Mood Swings, Anxiety

Remembering that sugar causes a release of the 'feel-good' hormone dopamine, you should expect some emotional reactions when you don't get your 'fix'. It will take a short while for your brain to adapt, so ride it out and don't worry too much about it. Letting your close co-workers know what you're doing and that you may be a little off-balance for a few days helps amazingly. Apologize in advance, explain what's up, and you'll have their support, assistance, and understanding. These symptoms are usually short-lived but they can return sporadically.

Fatigue & Body Aches

These are what have earned this group of reactions the nickname of 'flu'. General lethargy, mild muscle or joint aches, tiring easily, and even chills are the main symptoms. Treat yourself gently, nap if you can, and take it easy. It usually doesn't last more than 2-3 days and is usually mild. Skip your normal workout if you develop these symptoms until they've passed.

Sleep Changes

Although many people sleep a lot when detoxing from sugar, others experience some challenges to sleeping soundly. Insomnia is not uncommon, nor is difficulty staying asleep. If such problems crop up, avoid visual stimulation in the hour before going to bed, like TV or computer games. Try hot baths, chamomile tea, and reading instead. If the problem is persistent, try a magnesium supplement since this helps a lot of people. We all understand how difficult it is to lose a good night's sleep, but again this symptom will usually not last more than a few days.

Those are the things to be forewarned against when it comes to sugar withdrawal. A little knowledge can help you cope very well, and you may be one of the lucky few who experience no withdrawal symptoms at all. Just remember that there's really nothing wrong --- they're all signals that your body is working to put itself right again. Once the initial adjustment period has passed, you'll feel better, sleep better, think more clearly, and have more energy than ever before... and you'll start to drop some excess weight too!

CHAPTER V: BACK IN CONTROL IN 14 DAYS

You've done your homework and you're all set to start... so what now? Sugar detoxing has two main parts.

The first will jump-start your detox by having you go 'cold turkey', as they say. You'll not only cut out *all* sugar and sugar substitutes. You'll also be avoiding a number of other foods. Dairy and fruit contain their own forms of sugar, lactose and fructose, so they are off the menu for a few days and added back later in limited quantities. Grains, starches, and alcohol are quickly and easily metabolized into sugar, so they're out too.

Beginning with Day 4, many of these foods will be gradually brought back onto the menu and your meals will have much more variety. Many of these dishes and techniques may become part of your permanent recipe collection, whatever eating plan you choose to follow once you've completed your detox.

Your Meal Plan: 3-day super detox plus 3 week menu

Hopefully, you've made your sugar detox exit plan. You can use the guidelines from that eating protocol to customize both the general meal plan given here and the recipes. If you intend to stay low carb, for instance, you won't want to add back into your meals the fruits and grains that are gradually re-introduced in the second and third weeks. Instead, substitute low carbohydrate alternatives and increase the fats substantially. Sub out the oatmeal breakfasts for scotch eggs. Your menu for the last week should be very close to the diet you intend to continue eating, so make sure to begin to tailor the meals to your exit plan and add in any meals from that diet plan that you'd like to try.

Below are lists of the 'approved' foods for the Jump Start. Add-ins are indicated week by week.

Approved Foods and Beverages

Beverages	Proteins	Veggies	Fruit	Condiments	Other
1 cup black coffee	Chicken Turkey	Arugula Asparagus Bok Choy	Lemon Lime	Vinegar: Red Wine Balsamic Apple Cider	Nuts: up to 1 oz. twice a day
green or herbal tea (No limit)	Eggs	Broccoli Brussels sprouts		Butter, Coconut Oil, Olive Oil	Herbs & Spices (No Limit)
64 oz. water	Fish Shellfish	Cabbage, Cauliflower Celery			
	Tofu	Cucumbers Kale Lettuce			
		Olives Mushroom Peppers			
		Spinach Zucchini			

Week One Add-ins (daily): 1 additional cup of coffee, 1 serving dairy, 1 apple, grass-fed or lean beef, carrots, squash,

& tomatoes

Week Two Add-ins (daily): 1 additional dairy, berries, cantaloupe, grapefruit, up to 3 glasses of red wine per week

Week Three Add-ins: cherries, grapes, peaches, oranges, nectarines, oatmeal, whole grains (barley, buckwheat), dark chocolate (85% cacao or more)

Jump Start (Days 1-3)

...will begin the detoxifying process. Your sugar intake will be strictly limited, and you may begin to feel withdrawal effects by Day 2. This is the part that may require the most will power! Use the time to shop ahead for future meals and to solidify your 'exit plan' diet. The menu is the same for all 3 days.

For these 3 days, you <u>may not have</u>: sugars [including 'natural' and/or hidden sugars], artificial sweeteners, dairy, fruit, grains, starches, or alcohol.

Breakfast:
- 1 cup unsweetened coffee or green tea
- 3 eggs [cooked your way] with approved veggies OR a protein shake (no fruit or sugar)
- Water with fresh lemon or lime

Snacks [AM & PM]:
- 1 oz. nuts

Lunch:
- up to 6 oz. protein of choice [chicken, turkey, fish, shellfish, or tofu]
- small salad with homemade sugarless dressing

Dinner:
- up to 8 oz. protein of choice [same list as lunch]

- steamed approved veggies
- small salad with homemade sugarless dressing

**All recipes are included with meal plan

Day 4
Breakfast: Gussied-Up Greek Yogurt
Lunch: Chicken Mushroom Salad
Dinner: Roasted Shrimp with Garlic

Day 5
Breakfast: 3-Bite Frittatas
Lunch: Roasted Asparagus Soup with a small salad
Dinner: Pulled Garlic Pork with Cauli-Rice

Day 6
Breakfast: Protein Shake or Bulletproof Coffee®
Lunch: Pulled Pork [as lettuce wrap, taco, or on a salad]
Dinner: Roasted Asparagus Soup &Chicken with Artichoke and Olives

Day 7:
Breakfast: 3-Bite Frittatas
Lunch: Simple Chicken Soup & a small salad
Dinner: Poached Fish with Roasted Veggies

Day 8:
Breakfast: Gussied-Up Greek Yogurt
Lunch: Avocado Egg Salad [as lettuce wrap,taco, or on a salad]
Dinner: Spaghetti Squash & Meatballs

Day 9:
Breakfast: Scotch Eggs
Lunch: Chicken Salad [as lettuce wrap, taco, or on a salad]
Dinner: Spring Rolls with Nut Sauce

Day 10:

Breakfast: Protein Shake, Smoothie, or bulletproof coffee
Lunch: Salad with leftover Spring Rolls or Meatballs
Dinner: Stuffed Steak with Roasted Sprouts & Mushrooms

Day 11:
Breakfast: 3-Egg Omelet
Lunch: 3-Bean Chili
Dinner: Apple & Olive Spinach Salad

Day 12:
Breakfast: Berry Greek Yogurt
Lunch: Green Chili Salmon Muffins with a small salad
Dinner: Moroccan Chicken with Lemon

Day 13:
Breakfast: Ham-arrito
Lunch: CauliTabbouleh
Dinner: Wasabi Crab Cakes

Day 14:
Breakfast: 3-Bite Frittatas
Lunch: Tuna Salad [as lettuce wrap, taco, or on a salad]
Dinner: Chicken Quick Stir Fry

10-Day Bonus Meal Plans

Day 15:
Breakfast: Sausage Breakfast Casserole
Lunch: Waldorf Chicken Salad
Dinner: Poached Fish with Roasted Veggies

Day 16:
Breakfast: Protein Shake, Smoothie, or bulletproof coffee
Lunch: Small Salad with Devilled Eggs and/or 3-Bite Frittatas
Dinner: Sausage Red Curry Stroganoff

Day 17:

Breakfast: Sausage Breakfast Casserole
Lunch: Mushroom-Broccoli Soup with Devilled Eggs and/or 3-Bite Frittatas
Dinner: Seafood Balls with Homemade Tartar Sauce

Day 18:
Breakfast: Baked Oatmeal
Lunch: Orange-Berry Salad
Dinner: Pulled Pork

Day 19:
Breakfast: 3 Eggs Your Way
Lunch: Chili con Carne
Dinner: Spring Rolls with Pulled Pork

Day 20:
Breakfast: Ham-arrito
Lunch: Spring Rolls or Chili
Dinner: Stuffed Steak with Roasted Veggies

Day 21:
Breakfast: Baked Oatmeal
Lunch: Cobb Salad
Dinner: Spaghetti Squash and Meatballs

Day 22:
Breakfast: Gussied-Up Greek Yogurt
Lunch: Squash Soup with Devilled Eggs & salad
Dinner: 3-Bean Chili

Day 23:
Breakfast: Scotch Eggs
Lunch: Tuna Salad [as lettuce wrap, taco, or on a salad]
Dinner: Antipasto Kabobs

Day 24:
Breakfast: Oat Cakes
Lunch: Tabbouleh
Dinner: Poached Fish with Veggies

CHAPTER VI: LOW-SUGAR LIVING

Most of these recipes have 'planned leftovers' to give you a quick protein to use for lunches. Also plan ahead and cook when you have the time since many dishes freeze well. Slow cookers are great for making soups and for cooking chicken or turkey in advance. Using skin-on bone-in poultry will give you the best flavor as well as saving you money. An immersion (or stick) blender is the easiest way to make good mayonnaise and creamy soups/sauces, so consider purchasing one if you don't already have one.

Try a variety of herbal teas, hot or iced, to add some variety to your diet as well. Flavored liquid stevia is also a great way to vary the taste of beverages or plain yogurt without added or unwanted ingredients. If your options on that are limited locally, you can find a wide variety of flavors on Amazon.com and a bottle will last a long time.

Let's start with some salad dressings and grain/pasta substitutes that you'll use in other recipes.

Mayo

With a one-pint wide-mouth Mason jar and an immersion blender, this recipe is almost foolproof. If it somehow doesn't emulsify for you, turn it into salad dressing!

Ingredients:
- 1 large or extra-large egg
- 2-3 tsp. vinegar (or fresh lemon or lime juice)
- ¼ tsp. sea salt
- 1 c. extra light olive oil

Add all ingredients to a wide-mouth glass jar. [Make sure your blender will fit!] Let ingredients sit until the egg in on the bottom of the jar, usually only a few seconds. Put your blender in the jar with the head touching the bottom of the jar. *Without moving the blender*, turn it on and hold it in place for 20 seconds. You should see the mixture turning into mayo. After 20 seconds, move the blender upwards and around to make sure all the oil is blended in. Store the mayo in an airtight container and refrigerate for up to 2 weeks.

You can flavor the mayo by adding 2 T. Dijon mustard, some minced garlic, horseradish, or whatever takes your fancy. Be creative!

Tartar Sauce

Mix ¾ c mayo with 3 T pickle relish, ¼ tsp. garlic powder, juice from ½ lemon, and salt (to taste).

Salad Dressings

Just a few ideas to get you started! Make them right in a storage jar using an immersion blender and store refrigerated. Many are best if made the day before to let the flavors meld.

Basic Vinaigrette: 1 1/2 cextra virgin olive oil; 1/2 c apple cider vinegar; 2-4 cloves of garlic (minced); 1 tsp. dried oregano; 2 tsp. dried parsley; salt and pepper to taste

Vinaigrette Variations: replace the apple cider vinegar with lemon, lime, or orange juice or crushed blueberries/raspberries; substitute different spices; add a few finely diced nuts

Greek Dressing: 3/4 c olive oil; 1 c red wine vinegar; 2 tsp. each of garlic powder, dried oregano, and dried basil; 1 1/2 tsp. each of onion powder and black pepper; 1 tsp. salt; 2 tsp. Dijon mustard; 1 1/2 T lemon juice

Dijon Dressing: ½ c extra virgin olive oil; 2 T red wine vinegar; 3 T finely chopped shallots; 1 T plus 2 tsp. Dijon mustard; 1 tsp. salt; ½ tsp. freshly ground black pepper

Ginger-Miso Dressing: 4T miso; 4T olive oil; 2 tsp. lemon juice; 2T grated ginger; 1/2 c water

Sweet Apple Dressing: 1/4 cmayo; 1 T unsweetened apple sauce; 1/2 garlic clove, minced; 2 1/2 tsp. apple cider vinegar; just less than 1 tsp. ground mustard

Cauliflower Rice

This substitute for rice is used in many low carb recipes and offers a very healthy and inexpensive alternative to grains. Use it to replace rice in any recipe or as a base under other dishes. It keeps up to 3 days in the fridge and up to 2 months in the freezer, so prep it ahead of time.

Directions:
1. First remove all the green from the cauliflower, and cut it into chunks. Use a food processor to pulse it into rice (or couscous) sized bits, or you can use a cheese grater and do it by hand.
2. The easiest way to cook the cauli rice is the microwave. Put the cauli rice in a microwave-safe bowl, cover it with plastic wrap, and zap it for 3 minutes on High (if it's frozen, allow 4 minutes). Season with salt *after cooking* or it will get soggy.
3. You can also stir fry the cauli rice in a sauté pan with a little olive oil, which gives it a nice flavor but also makes it a little clumpy. Roasting gives the 'rice' the best texture. Spread it in a thin layer on a baking sheet, drizzle with just a little olive oil, and cook at 350 degrees for about 12 minutes, stirring halfway through the cooking time.

Faux Tortillas

These cauliflower-based tortillas provide a non-grain option for wraps. If you're not a fan of lettuce/cabbage wraps, give these a try. Cauliflower may become your new best friend as a grain replacement food!

Ingredients:
- 3 packed cups uncooked, riced cauliflower
- 6 egg whites
- Sea salt

Directions:
1. Grate the cauliflower very fine in a food processor or by hand. In a microwave- safe large bowl, put three packed cups of the grated cauliflower. Microwave it for 3 minutes; then, stir well and microwave it for another 2 minutes. Spread the cauliflower on a clean kitchen towel, roll it up, and twist to wring all the water out. Be careful not to burn yourself! Spread the cauliflower on a baking sheet and refrigerate it. Once it's cooled and ready to use, preheat the oven to 350 degrees F. and cover a baking sheet with parchment.
2. In a large bowl, combine the cauliflower, the egg whites, and salt to taste. Mix well with a spoon. It may seem a little runny, but spoon it onto the parchment, making circles about 8 inches in diameter. Bake the tortillas for about 10 minutes and then flip them and bake for another 6-7 minutes. Cool them flat on a wire rack. Before using, give the tortillas a minute per side in a hot fry pan.

Veggie Noodles

Spaghetti squash is the classic veggie noodle. Once the squash is cooked, the insides can be 'shredded out' with a fork into long pasta-like noodles. You can, however, make 'noodles' from any hard vegetable. Zucchini is particularly popular due to its mild taste, and the result is often referred to as 'zoodles'. Carrots, parsnips, asparagus, and even broccoli stems work well. Many veggie noodles even pass the 'kid test'!

Directions:
1. If you don't have a spiralizer, which produces long beautiful noodles, use a box grater or even a peeler to cut long thin strips of veggies. Steam them until they turn soft. Season to taste and enjoy!

Gussied-Up Greek Yogurt

Directions:

1. Start with whole milk [full fat] plain Greek yogurt. This can sometimes be hard to find, and you may need to buy a large container and divide out the servings.
2. Add up to 1 T nuts, cinnamon, and a few drops of vanilla extract. Stir well.
3. You may vary the nuts, spices, and extracts to suit yourself and to create very different flavors. I'm particularly fond of walnuts with a just a little maple extract. Liquid stevia can help to take the tart edge off, especially if you're used to commercial yogurt that's highly sweetened. Just use a drop or two! Remember, you don't want it to taste sweet, just not quite so sour!

Chicken Mushroom Salad

A great, hearty salad, sometimes called 'Wedding Salad', that you can prep the night before and enjoy cold (or heated) the next day. Don't leave out the pickles because they really give it a spark!

Ingredients:
- 1 lb. chicken, cooked and diced
- ¾ lb. mushrooms, diced
- 1 lg. carrot, grated
- 1 small onion, finely diced
- 2 T. mayo
- 5-6 baby dill pickles, finely diced
- Salt & Pepper to taste

Directions:
1. Put the diced chicken in a large bowl. Using a store-cooked rotisserie chicken is a real time saver, or you can cook chicken overnight in the slow cooker beforehand.
2. Sauté mushrooms until moisture is cooked out, then season with salt and pepper. Cook until browned. Add to chicken in the bowl.
3. Cook the carrots and onion in oil until softened. Add them to the bowl.
4. Add the diced dills to the salad. Mix ingredients together with the mayo. Add more or less mayo to taste.

Roasted Shrimp with Garlic

This is a quick and easy recipe that tastes very much like Shrimp Scampi. Serve over zucchini noodles, which can be steamed or raw, or cauli-rice.

Ingredients:
- 8 oz. peeled, deveined shrimp
- 2 T melted butter
- 2 T coconut or olive oil
- 2 garlic cloves, minced
- 1 lemon
- ¼ tsp. salt
- freshly ground black pepper (to taste)

Directions:
1. Preheat oven to 400 degrees.
2. Zest and juice the lemon, and then combine everything in a baking dish.
3. Cook in the oven for 8-10 minutes until shrimp are cooked. Turn the shrimp midway through the cooking time.

3-Bite Frittatas

These little gems are easy, delicious, and great for using up leftovers. Make several batches at once (they freeze well) to have on hand for a quick breakfast, snack, or light lunch/dinner with a salad. Add ham, olives, or whatever you like to vary the taste.

Ingredients:
- 8 eggs
- 2 c chopped veggies or meat
- 2 T. fresh herbs of choice
- a pinch of salt & pepper

Directions:
1. Preheat oven to 375 degrees and lightly grease a 12-cup muffin tin.
2. Beat the eggs, herbs, and salt/pepper in a large bowl until frothy.
3. Pour into the muffin cups, dividing evenly.
4. Add the chopped veggies/meat to each cup.
5. Bake for 10 minutes until a toothpick comes out clean and the frittatas are a little browned on top.
6. Let cool a bit before removing from pan.

Roasted Asparagus Soup

The unique taste of this soup is sure to please, and it keeps and reheats well. Roasting is a great way to change up the taste of a vegetable, and the avocado adds richness!

Ingredients:
- 12 oz. asparagus
- 1 tsp. minced garlic
- 1 T. olive oil
- 2 c. broth [chicken, bone, or veggie]
- 1 avocado, peeled and cubed
- ½ lemon, juiced
- 1 T. butter
- salt& pepper (to taste)

Directions:
1. Preheat oven to 425 degrees.
2. Toss the asparagus with the oil and garlic. Add salt/pepper to taste. Place in a baking pan and roast for about 10 minutes
3. Put the asparagus in a blender along with the remaining ingredients and puree until smooth.
4. Add water or broth to thin to your preferred consistency, and add salt & pepper to taste.
5. If needed, gently reheat.

Pulled Garlic Pork with Cauli-Rice [slow cooker]

This is a really easy slow cooker recipe that makes your cauli rice right along with the meat. Make sure to save some of the pork for tomorrow's lunch!

Ingredients:
- 2 lb. pork rump roast
- 6 cloves garlic, peeled
- 2 heads cauliflower, stemmed and grated [see Cauli Rice recipe]
- 1 c chicken broth
- 1 tsp. cumin
- 1 tsp. salt
- ½ tsp. black pepper

Directions:
1. Put the riced cauliflower into the slow cooker. Add 3 cloves of the garlic, the cumin, and the salt and pepper.
2. Make three one-inch slits into the pork roast and insert a garlic clove into each. Put the roast into the slow cooker on top of the riced cauliflower.
3. Cook on Low 8-10 hours. Use two forks to shred the meat.

Protein Shake

Directions:
1. Choose a whey protein powder carefully to avoid hidden sugars or artificial sweeteners.
2. Mix it with 6 oz. full-fat Greek yogurt. From there, you can add almond or peanut butter, nuts, fresh or frozen unsweetened berries, chia or hemp seeds, and even spinach or kale for your additional nutrients and flavors.
3. Blend until smooth, and then thin to your preferred consistency with unsweetened almond or coconut milk.

Bulletproof Coffee®

You can also use green tea for this beverage, but it's not as effective, especially for weight loss. Start with the lowest amount of butter and coconut oil. If you want to have this often for breakfast, gradually increase the amount of butter and coconut oil you use.

Ingredients:
- 2 cups low-toxin brewed coffee [or green tea]
- 1-2 T grass-fed butter
- 1-2 T coconut oil

Directions:
1. While the coffee is brewing, put hot water in a glass blender to pre-heat it. When you're ready to make your coffee, empty the water.
2. Put all the ingredients into the blender.
3. Put the lid on with a kitchen towel over it. Holding the lid down with your hand (and the towel), blend the beverage until you have a nice froth on the top. [You can use an immersion or hand blender but it won't mix as quite as well.]
4. Pour into a mug and drink somewhat slowly to allow time for your system to process the oils.

Chicken with Artichokes and Olives [slow cooker]

Another crockpot meal with lots of flavor and flair! After cooking, you can use a little brown rice flour or tapioca flour to thicken the juice into a tasty sauce. Also, throw in a few extra pieces of chicken to cook now for use later in the week in soup and chicken salad.

Ingredients:
- 4 chicken breasts
- 14 oz. can of artichoke hearts, drained
- 14 oz. can of pitted olives, drained [any type of olive you like]
- 1 onion, chopped
- ½ c white wine
- 1 c chicken stock
- 1 tsp. dried thyme
- 1 garlic clove, minced
- ¼ tsp. each of salt & pepper
- 2 T capers [if you have them]

Directions:
1. Mix all ingredients into the slow cooker. Cover and cook on low for 7-8 hours until chicken is done all the way through.

Simple Chicken Soup

This recipe is super quick if you have some chicken already cooked and ready to use. Otherwise, cook your chicken in water with some carrots, onion, and celery for about 30 minutes and let cool enough to shred or chop. Strain the broth.

Ingredients:
- 3 carrots, peeled and thinly sliced
- 2 stalks of celery, thinly sliced
- 1-2 qt. chicken broth
- uncooked veggie noodles
- chicken, chopped or shredded

Directions:
1. Simmer carrots and celery in the chicken broth until tender.
2. Add veggie noodles and chicken, and cook until the noodles have softened.

Poached Fish

Poaching keeps fish moist and tender, and it's quick to do. This method is particularly good with low fat fish such as cod, tilapia, or halibut. Score the skin side to keep the fish from curling up as it cooks.

Ingredients:
- 1 leek or shallot, shredded or diced
- 1 bay leaf
- 4 slices of lemon
- 1 T butter
- a few black peppercorns
- pinch of salt
- 4 portions of fish
- olive oil or butter, to garnish

Directions:
1. Choose a deep pot that is large enough for all your fish to lie flat. Put everything except the fish in the pot, add 6 cups water, bring to a boil, and reduce heat and simmer for 20-30 minutes.
2. Further reduce heat and add the fish. It should be at least two-thirds covered with liquid. Add water if needed.
3. Bring back to a boil, and then turn off the heat completely. Cover and let steam on the stovetop for 7-10 minutes until fish is opaque and flaky.
4. Carefully remove the fish and serve drizzled with a little olive oil or butter.

Roasted Veggies

Vegetables are terrific when they're roasted, and it's a quick easy way to prepare them. Asparagus, broccoli, cauliflower, and Brussels sprouts have a different flavor when they're not steamed, and you can turn carrots, parsnips, and zucchini into 'faux fries'. Add whatever herbs and spices you'd like!

Directions:
1. Preheat oven to 425 degrees.
2. Toss the vegetables with coconut or olive oil. Add salt/pepper, herbs, spices, or garlic to taste. Place on a baking sheet and roast for about 10 minutes or until the vegetables reach the doneness you like.

Avocado Egg Salad

The avocado adds richness and healthy fats to this egg salad, and you can leave out the cayenne pepper if you prefer it milder. This recipe is one you'll reach for long after finishing the Sugar Detox!

Ingredients:
- 8 large hard-boiled eggs, chopped
- 1/2 c mayonnaise
- 1/2 c salsa
- 1/2 c onion, finely chopped
- 1/2 c celery, finely chopped
- 1 large avocado
- 2 T lime juice
- salt and pepper, to taste
- cayenne pepper, to taste

Directions:
1. Cut the avocado in half, remove the pit, and scoop out the flesh into a bowl. Mash the avocado with the lime juice.
2. Add the mayo, salsa, onion, and celery and mix well.
3. Gently stir the chopped eggs into the mixture. Season to taste with salt, pepper, and cayenne. Refrigerate before eating to allow the flavors to combine nicely.

Spaghetti Squash & Meatballs

With or without tomato sauce, this is a hearty and healthy meal that's also very kid-friendly. Sprinkle with a little grated Parmesan cheese and enjoy, but save some meatballs for lunches later.

Ingredients:
- 1 large spaghetti squash
- 2 lb. ground meat [mix beef, pork, chicken, or turkey]
- 1 egg
- 2 T minced chives
- 2 T minced basil
- 2-3 garlic cloves, minced
- ½ onion, chopped
- ½ c minced sun-dried tomatoes
- 2 tsp. salt
- 1 tsp. black pepper

Directions:
1. Cut the stem end off the squash so it will stand on end. Then carefully cut the squash in half lengthwise. Carefully clean out the seeds and discard them.
2. Place the squash cut-side down in a microwave-safe dish. Add about an inch of water. Microwave for approximately 12 minutes until you can poke a fork into it easily. Let cool until it's easy to handle, and use a fork to scrape out the insides into spaghetti-like noodles. [To cook in the oven, place the squash cut-side down on a baking sheet. Bake at 375 degrees for about 40 minutes.] Salt to taste.
3. In a large bowl, combine all the other ingredients, mixing well. Form into small balls. Fry in coconut oil (in batches) until browned and cooked through or cook the meatballs in the oven at 350 degrees for 15-20 minutes or until done.

Scotch Eggs

Portable eggs and sausage is hard to beat! Make lots of these to have for breakfasts, lunches, and very hearty snacks. Season the sausage with whatever herbs and spices you'd like, or try using some chorizo mixed in for a different taste.

Ingredients:
- 8 eggs, hard boiled and peeled
- 2 lbs. bulk pork sausage
- herbs and spices to taste

Directions:
1. Preheat oven to 375 degrees and get out a muffin pan.
2. Lay a piece of plastic wrap on your workspace and place about and eighth of the sausage on it. Use your hands to make a circular shape about ½ inch thick. (You may want to get this step ready now for all your eggs.)
3. Place one egg in the center of the sausage patty you've created. Put your hand under the plastic wrap and pick it all up. Use your hand (and the plastic) to wrap the sausage completely around the egg, sealing it inside the meat. Finish shaping with your bare hands if you need to. Place each wrapped egg as it's finished into a cup of a muffin pan.
4. Bake for about 25 minutes, pull out and carefully drain the fat, and return to oven for another 5-10 minutes. You want your sausage cooked all the way through.
5. Remove the eggs from the pan and let them cool on a wire rack for 5-10 minutes.
6. Enjoy the scotch eggs hot or cold. They keep for a couple of days in the fridge, but you can freeze the extras.

Chicken Salad

An easy lunch classic that you can eat by itself, on a salad, or wrap in a cauli-tortilla! Use either avocado or mayo to change up the taste. This is a small recipe for 2 servings so double or triple as you will.

Ingredients:
- 1 c diced or shredded chicken
- 1 stalk celery
- 1 small carrot
- 1 scallion
- ½ apple
- 1 T Dijon mustard
- 1 tsp. capers
- salt and pepper (to taste)
- ½ avocado (mashed with 1 tsp. lemon juice) **or** mayo (to hold salad together)

Directions:
1. Dice the celery, carrot, scallion, and apple. Mix them together with the chicken and capers in a bowl.
2. Stir in your avocado mix or mayo. Mix the mustard, and add salt and pepper.

Spring Rolls with Nut Sauce

This Asian 'portable salad' is simple to make and a wonderful way to use up leftovers as well. Look for the rice paper rolls/wrappers near the tofu in your market, with the ethnic foods, or in an Asian market. Keep any leftover spring rolls refrigerated for lunch tomorrow.

Ingredients:
- Rice Paper Rolls/Wrappers
- Any cooked meat or fish
- Vegetables such as cabbage, carrots, bean sprouts, avocado, zucchini
- Herbs such as cilantro, basil, or mint

Directions:
1. Slice your filling ingredients very thinly or julienne them.
2. Fill a large bowl with warm (not hot) water. Dip a rice paper completely into the water, and then place it on your worktop.
3. Arrange your filling in the center of the rice paper, leaving a couple of inches around the edges. You'll need the unfilled area for the wrapping process so don't overfill each one!
4. Fold the top part of the rice paper down over the ingredients. Then fold the two sides in over the middle. Tidy up any stray filling, and then roll the top portion towards you, trying to keep a nice tight roll. Seal the edge with a little water to close it up.
5. Slice the spring roll in half to serve.

Nut Sauce

Whisk all ingredients until well combined. Use as a dipping sauce for your homemade spring rolls or as a dressing for salads.
- ½ c peanut or almond butter
- ¼ c water

- 2 T tamari [liquid aminos or coconut aminos] or soy sauce
- sprinkle of red pepper flakes

Stuffed Steak

This is an elegant dish, quite suitable for guests. You can vary the stuffing ingredients and herbs to get very different tastes.

Ingredients:
- 3 lb. top round or flank steak
- 1 c chopped mushrooms
- 1 shallot, chopped
- ¼ c chopped ham
- 1 T parsley
- ½ tsp. dried thyme

Directions:
1. Combine the mushrooms, shallot, and ham in a sauté pan with a little oil. Cook covered for 5 minutes or until mushrooms are soft. Stir in the herbs and remove from the heat.
2. Make a slit in the steak from one side to form a large pocket. Fill with the cooled stuffing mixture and close the slit with toothpicks (or a turkey trussing kit if you have one).
3. Brush the steak lightly with oil and broil, turning once, for 5-10 minutes a side depending how well you like it done. Slice into half-inch thick servings.

3-Bean Chili [slow cooker]

A hearty vegetarian chili that's easy to cook overnight with your crockpot. On the stovetop, this chili will need to simmer for at least an hour to marry the flavors.

Ingredients:
- 2 red bell peppers, cleaned and diced
- 1 c onion, chopped
- 2 tsp. ground cumin
- 1 tsp. crushed red pepper
- 1 tsp. paprika
- ¼ tsp. salt
- 4 cloves of garlic, thinly sliced
- 2 c vegetable broth
- 1 ½ c butternut squash, peeled and cubed
- 28 oz. can no-salt-added diced tomatoes (with liquid)
- 15 oz. can pinto beans, rinsed and drained
- 15 oz. can cannellini beans, rinsed and drained
- 15 oz. can red kidney beans, rinsed and drained
- (as garnish) ½ cup green onions, thinly sliced

Directions:
1. Combine everything in the crock of the slow cooker. Stir to mix well.
2. Cover and cook for 7-12 hours on Low.

Apple & Olive Spinach Salad

The unusual pairing of apples with green olives gives this salad a delicious sweet and salty tang. The recipe serves only one, so multiply it out, and top it off with some sweet apple dressing.

Ingredients:
- fresh spinach
- ½ apple
- ½ avocado
- 8 pitted green olives
- Protein of choice: chicken breast or shrimp
- slivered almonds to garnish

Directions:
Chop all ingredients and toss together with the spinach leaves.Garnish with a sprinkle of almonds. Serve drizzled with sweet apple dressing.

Green Chili Salmon Muffins

These little fish loaves are tasty, very portable, and easy to heat in the microwave for a quick lunch. They use almond flour, which you can find in the organic baking section in many large supermarkets. Double or triple the recipe and freeze after baking.

Ingredients:
- 1 lb. salmon filets, skin removed [or equivalent of canned salmon]
- 1 stalk celery, chopped
- ½ onion, chopped
- 1 egg
- 1 4-oz. can diced green chilies
- ¼ cup almond flour
- 1 tsp. garlic powder
- 1 tsp. chipotle chili powder
- 1/2 T parsley
- Salt and pepper to taste

Directions:
1. Grease the cups on a muffin pan and preheat oven to 350 degrees.
2. Put all the ingredients in a food processor and blend until well mixed.
3. Place a ¼ cup of mixture into each muffin cup, and bake for 30-35 minutes until they are just beginning to brown on the edges.

Moroccan Chicken with Lemon

You'll need a preserved lemon for this one, so look in the baking or ethnic section of your market. This is terrific served over cauli-rice!

Ingredients:
- 1 batch spice mix (below)
- 1 ½ lbs. chicken pieces, bone-in and skin-on
- 1 T olive or coconut oil
- 2 cloves garlic, minced
- 1 yellow onion, sliced
- 1 preserved lemon, rinsed and thinly sliced
- ½ c pitted green olives, chopped
- ¼ c raisins
- ½ c water
- ¼ c cilantro or parsley, chopped (garnish)

Directions:
1. Make sure your chicken pieces are dry, and then rub them with the spice mix.
2. Heat the oil in a saucepan on medium. Begin browning the chicken, turning as needed.
3. Add the garlic and onion to the pan and cook until golden.
4. Add in the sliced lemon, olives, raisins, and water. Cover and simmer for 15 minutes or until chicken is cooked through.
5. Serve spooned over cauli-rice and sprinkled with cilantro or parsley.

Spice Mix

1 tsp. paprika, ½ tsp. each of cumin, ginger, and turmeric, ¼ tsp. cinnamon, 1/8 tsp. black pepper. Combine and mix well.

Ham-arrito

This is a great take on a breakfast burrito that uses ham instead of tortillas.

Directions:
1. If the ham is very thinly sliced, you'll need to use two or three slices so it doesn't break.
2. Make scrambled eggs with leftover cooked veggies or fresh ones like bell peppers, and don't forget extras like black olives.
3. Place a scoop of your cooked egg scramble in the middle of the ham.
4. Fold the top in, then the sides, and roll it up. You can heat the whole thing afterwards or not, your call.
5. Store any extras tightly wrapped in plastic film to reheat in the microwave.

CauliTabbouleh

Tabbouleh is a traditional Middle Eastern salad, prepared here with cauliflower to avoid the grains. Fresh mint adds a unique flavor.

Ingredients:
- 2 heads of cauliflower, cleaned and riced
- 1 ½ c fresh flat-leaf parsley, cut in pieces
- ½ c fresh mint, cut in pieces
- 3 tomatoes, diced
- 6 T olive oil
- 2 T lemon juice
- 2 cloves garlic, minced
- salt and fresh-ground pepper (to taste)

Directions:
1. Put the grated cauliflower into a large bowl. Add in the parsley, mint, and tomato and mix well. Season with salt and pepper to taste.
2. Whisk together the oil, lemon juice, and garlic. Drizzle all of it over the salad.
3. Toss the salad to distribute the dressing evenly.

Wasabi Crab Cakes

The unusual combination of unsweetened coconut and almond flour gives these crab cakes a great and grain-free crunch. The wasabi and avocado sauce is both spicy and creamy. Together these make for a quick and delicious meal.

Ingredients:
- 1 lb. lump crabmeat, drained
- 3 green onions, finely sliced
- ¼ c diced red bell pepper,
- 2 egg yolks
- ½ tsp. garlic powder
- ½ tsp. onion powder
- ☐ c mayo
- ¼ tsp. sea salt
- ¼ tsp. black pepper
- dash of red pepper
- ☐ c blanched almond flour
- ☐ c unsweetened shredded coconut
- 2 T coconut oil

Directions:
1. In a large bowl, combine crab, veggies, egg yolks, and the spices and mix well. Form them into small patties and refrigerate for 15 minutes or so.
2. In a dish or plate, mix the almond flour and the coconut. Heat the oil in a large fry pan on high.
3. Press both sides of the crab cakes into the coconut-flour mixture, coating them. Shake off any excess, and then fry the crab cakes for about 4 minutes per side. They should be nicely browned.
4. Serve with wasabi sauce [below] drizzled or spooned on top.

Wasabi Sauce

Use a blender to combine the following ingredients until smooth:

- 1 avocado, peeled, pitted, and cubed
- 1 T mayonnaise
- 2 tsp. wasabi paste
- ⅓ c water
- 1 T coconut aminos, liquid aminos, or tamari
- 1 T rice vinegar
- dash of sea salt

Tuna Salad

Add some carrot, avocado, and pickle for variety and some herbs and spices to liven it up.

Chicken Quick Stir Fry

This is a great recipe to whip up very quickly, especially if you have some chicken already cooked and some leftover vegetables. Try it with Brussels sprouts---yum!

Ingredients:
- 1 lb. sliced mushrooms
- 2 heads broccoli, cleaned and cut up
- 1 whole onion, sliced
- 1 garlic clove, minced
- 1/4 c chicken broth
- 2 chicken breasts, cut into bite-sized pieces
- 2 Tcoconut aminos
- salt&pepper (to taste)
- 2 tablespoons vegetable oil

Directions:
1. Heat oil in wok or large fry pan over medium-low heat.
2. Cook chicken, stirring and turning frequently, until browned.
3. Add onion and garlic and cook until onion is translucent and caramelized.
4. Add all the remaining ingredients. Cover and cook until the veggies are done. Add a little more water, if needed. It should have a little broth.
5. Serve with or over cauli-rice.

Sausage Breakfast Casserole

Spinach and cauliflower 'grits' turn this into a hearty way to start your day. Make it ahead and just heat a serving in the microwave. If you have stored some 'riced' cauliflower, this is really quick to mix up.

Ingredients:
- 1 head cauliflower, cleaned and grated
- 1 lb. bulk sausage
- 5 c fresh spinach
- 6 oz. full-fat coconut milk
- 4 eggs, lightly beaten
- juice from one lemon
- 2 tsp. salt
- 2 tsp. garlic powder
- ½ tsp. red pepper flakes

Directions:
1. Preheat oven to 350 degrees, and grease a 9 by 13 baking dish.
2. Heat 2-3 T coconut oil (or bacon grease) in a large skillet. Sauté the cauli bits until they're tender. Let them sit and cool, stirring from time to time.
3. Cook the sausage in the fry pan until crumbly. Add the spinach into the pan and cook until wilted.
4. In a large bowl, stir together the coconut milk and eggs. Add in the spinach-sausage mixture and stir well. Finally add in the seasonings and the cauli 'grits'.
5. Spread your mixture into the baking pan. Bake for about 45 minutes until the center is set.

Waldorf Chicken Salad

This will use up your fruit allotment for the day but it's my favorite version of chicken salad ... and it's really easy! Double or triple this recipe as desired.

Ingredients:
- 2 cups chicken, cooked and cubed/shredded
- ½ sweet red apple, diced [red delicious]
- ½ tart green apple, diced [granny smith]
- 1 c seedless grapes, halved
- ½ c walnuts, chopped
- mayo(to taste)

Directions
1. Combine all ingredients in a bowl and mix well.
2. Stir in mayo until your salad sticks together.

Devilled Eggs

Use your favorite recipe as long as it's sugar and grain free. Try using mashed avocado in place of the mayo for a nutrient boost.

Sausage Red Curry Stroganoff

This is an Asian 'take' on stroganoff that's quick, easy, spicy, and unique. Serve it hot over cauli-rice or veggie noodles.

Ingredients:
- 1 T butter
- 1 yellow onion, chopped
- 2 garlic cloves, minced
- 1 lb. spicy sausage, sliced
- 3 T tomato paste
- 1 tsp. Thai red curry powder or paste
- 1 c full-fat coconut milk
- ½ tsp. salt & black pepper (to taste)

Directions:
1. Melt the butter in a large fry pan over medium-high heat.
2. Add the onion and cook until it's translucent.
3. Add in the garlic and the sausage, reduce heat to medium, and cook about 7 minutes until sausage is cooked.
4. Stir in the remaining ingredients and simmer until thickened. Season to taste with salt and pepper.

Mushroom-Broccoli Soup

Thick, earthy, and very satisfying ... this soup will hit all your buttons! You may add more water if you want a thinner consistency.

Ingredients:
- 1 T coconut oil
- 1 onion, diced
- 2 garlic cloves, minced
- 1 tsp. red pepper flakes
- 2 lbs. broccoli florets [no stems]
- 2 tsp. lemon juice
- 6 oz. mushrooms, chopped

Directions:
1. Heat the coconut oil in a large saucepan or stockpot. Add the onion and cook until translucent.
2. Add in the garlic and the red pepper flakes and let cook for about a minute, and then add the broccoli. Cook for 3-5 minutes.
3. Add about ½ c water along with the lemon juice. Cover and steam for 5 minutes until broccoli is almost tender.
4. Add in the mushrooms and cook a few minutes more.
5. Use a blender or immersion blender to puree until fairly smooth and serve.

Seafood Balls

This recipe is very inexpensive to make and very kid-friendly. You can vary the fish to shrimp ratio to suit yourself, and this makes up well with cod, which is easy to find. Shape it into sticks if you choose, but rolling the balls is quicker! Th double breading makes these nice and crunchy.

Ingredients:
- 1 ½ lb. cod
- ½ lb. shrimp, shelled and cleaned
- juice from a half lemon
- 3 T parsley, chopped
- 2 T Old Bay seasoning
- 2 eggs
- 2 T homemade tartar sauce
- ½ c almond flour

[for the breading]
- 1 egg
- ½ c water
- 1 c almond flour
- 1 tsp. salt

Directions:
1. Combine all ingredients [except for the breading ones] in the large bowl of your food processor. Process to a paste.
2. Heat a couple of tablespoons of fat in a large fry pan over medium-high heat.
3. Whisk the egg and water in a small bowl. In another small bowl, thoroughly combine the almond flour and the salt.
4. Spoon out the fish mixture and shape it into small balls. Roll each one in the flour mixture until covered, then put it into the egg mix, and then roll it in the flour again.
5. In several batches, sauté the seafood balls in the fry

pan until crispy and browned, about 3 minutes a side.
6. Serve with homemade tartar sauce.

Baked Oatmeal

Baked oatmeal can be mixed up the evening before and baked in the morning very easily. Make it without the baking powder and refrigerate overnight. Stir in the baking powder in the morning, put in the pan, and bake. Keep the leftovers for quick breakfasts later ... if you can!

Ingredients:
- 2 c rolled oats [not instant]
- rounded ½ tsp. baking powder
- 1 tsp. cinnamon
- ½ tsp. nutmeg
- ½ c chopped nuts
- 1 ½ c unsweetened almond milk
- ½ c unsweetened applesauce
- 1 banana [or fruit of choice]

Directions:
1. Preheat oven to 350 degrees.
2. Leaving out the banana, mix al the other ingredients in a large bowl. It will be a very thick batter.
3. Pour or spread the batter into a greased baking dish.
4. Slice the banana and arrange the slices on top of the batter, pushing them slightly into the batter.
5. Bake for 30-35 minutes.

Orange-Berry Salad
This combination is a refreshing change from all vegetable salads. Fruit takes center stage, and make the dressing ahead for quick assembly at lunchtime!

Ingredients:
[for the dressing]
- 1 c raspberries, fresh or frozen
- 1 T lime juice
- 1 T extra-virgin olive oil
- 1 tsp. Dijon mustard
- ¼ tsp. salt
- ¼ c water

[for the salad]
- spinach, kale, or leafy greens of choice
- 1 orange
- sliced almonds
- black pepper

Directions:
1. Combine all dressing ingredients in a blender and mix until smooth. Add extra water if you'd like the dressing a little thinner.
2. Put your greens on a plate. Peel and cut the orange into chunks to put on top of your greens.
3. Sprinkle with almonds and a little black pepper. Drizzle with the dressing and enjoy!

Tomatillo Pulled Pork [slow cooker]

Tomatillos give this dish it's unique taste, but you can make it using any spicy salsa. It's slow cooked to impart maximum flavor and tenderness. Save some to sneak into your Spring Rolls tomorrow night!

Ingredients:
- 2 lb. pork shoulder roast
- 1 red onion, chopped
- 1 Poblano pepper, chopped
- 2 garlic cloves, minced
- 16 oz. tomatillo salsa or Spanish green sauce
- juice of ½ lime
- 3 T fresh oregano, chopped

Directions:
1. Put you onion, pepper, and garlic into the slow cooker.
2. Place the roast into the slow cooker and pour the tomatillo sauce over it. Add the lime juice.
3. Cover and cook 8-10 hours on low.
4. Shred the meat with two forks and mix in the fresh oregano.

Chili Con Carne

True Texas-style chili has no beans ... and Texans are serious about that! You can simmer this on the stovetop or transfer it to a crockpot for some slow melding of the flavors. Traditionally, it's served sprinkled with diced onions and a little grated cheddar. Adjust the seasonings, so it's just spicy enough for you.

Ingredients:
- 1 lb. ground beef
- 1 onion, chopped
- 2 garlic cloves, minced
- 1 tsp. dried oregano
- 1 tsp. ground cumin
- 6 tsp. chili powder
- 1 small can diced green chilies
- 3 dashes hot sauce
- 1 dash habanero sauce
- 24 oz. no-salt diced tomatoes
- 1 c water

Directions:
1. Using a Dutch oven or stockpot, cook your meat and onion over medium heat. Break the meat into small pieces. Add the garlic for a few minutes at the end of the cook time. [Use a fry pan if you plan to do the chili in a crockpot. After cooking, transfer everything from the pan to the slow cooker, even the fat.]
2. Add your dry seasonings and stir to coat the meat with them. Then add all the remaining ingredients. Bring to a boil, then lower the heat, cover, and simmer for at least an hour. [6-10 hours in the slow cooker]
3. Skim off the grease and serve.

Cobb Salad

Cobb salad is distinguished by having the ingredients in stripes across the top and by featuring corn, whether in kernels or those tiny corncobs. Feel free to change out ingredients or toss it up as you choose. I'll also leave the quantities in your hands.

Directions:
1. Use a mixture of romaine lettuce and spinach for the base of the salad.
2. Top with stripes of chopped tomato, hard-boiled egg, crispy bacon, cooked corn, and chopped avocado.
3. Top it all with Greek dressing and some feta or cheddar cheese.

Squash Soup [slow cooker]

This is a very traditional recipe, but play with spices and additions to make it all your own. The soup is blended smooth after cooking.

Ingredients:
- 1 large butternut squash, peeled, cleaned, and cubed
- 14 oz. full-fat coconut milk
- 2 c chicken stock
- 1 tart apple, peeled, cored, and cubed
- 2 carrots, peeled and sliced
- 1 tsp. cinnamon
- 1 tsp. nutmeg

Directions:
1. Put all ingredients into the slow cooker.
2. Cover and cook on low for 4-6 hours.
3. Blend using an immersion blender right in the crockpot, or transfer to a pre-warmed traditional blender.
4. Serve topped with a sprinkle of bacon bits.

Antipasto Kabobs

These are simple easy good bites that can also be served as an appetizer. Use any sort of sausage or smoked sausage you like, or go with salami or a mild pepperoni. It's a little antipasto tray on a stick!

Ingredients:
- 1 lb. cooked or smoked sausage, cut in one-inch pieces
- cherry tomatoes
- 14 oz. artichoke hearts, drained
- marinated mushrooms
- pitted olives of choice
- skewers

Directions:
1. Preheat oven to 350 degrees.
2. In a fry pan, brown both sides of the sausage slices in a little oil. Remove them from the pan and set aside.
3. In the same pan, lightly cook the cherry tomatoes for about a minute, until they get a little browned in spots. Remove from heat.
4. Make each kabob by threading an olive onto the skewer, followed by a mushroom, artichoke heart, tomato, and a piece of sausage. Lay each completed kabob in a baking dish.
5. Cover the baking dish with foil and put in the oven for about 10 minutes until the kabobs are warmed through.

Oat Cakes

This is a very versatile recipe that can be adjusted easily to make the cakes lighter like muffins or denser like scones. Chia seeds are the magic ingredients in these cakes, so pick some up if you haven't already. Add in any nuts, fruit, or spices you like!

Ingredients:
- ½ c rolled oats
- ½ c oat flour [use a blender or food processor to convert rolled oats to flour]
- 1 T chia seeds
- ¼ tsp. baking powder
- water

Directions:
1. First make a gel from the chia seeds. Place 1 T of chia seeds in ½ cup of water. Let them sit for about 20 minutes until the seeds swell up. Use less chia gel for denser cakes or scones and more for muffins.
2. Preheat oven to 375 degrees and lightly grease baking sheet or muffin tin.
3. In a large bowl, mix all ingredients including your add-ins. The resulting dough will be thick.
4. Drop the batter with a spoon onto a baking sheet, or shape it into balls or biscuits. Bake for about 10 minutes until a toothpick inserted in the middle comes out clean.
5. Cool on a wire rack and store tightly covered.

SWEET SUCCESS!

It's a little hard to believe the health and wellness problems caused by excess sugar. Our sweetness quotient has risen drastically over the past 100 years, and it's been killing us ... literally. Sugar and its evil cousins, artificial sweeteners, have been sneaking into our food supply more and more with each passing year, without our knowledge.

We've been carefully watching our fat consumption when we should have been learning the many various names for 'sugar'!

This book has given you the information you need to reclaim your grip on the reins of this run-away sugar wagon. By doing a sugar detox, you'll begin your journey back to natural good health. More importantly, you now know how to avoid being wrapped up in sugar's chains ever again! You know how to find sugar no matter what name it's hiding under, and how to control your consumption for optimal good health and longevity. Knowing what goes into your body gives you back the ultimate control over your body.

As you've read, this is not a 'no sugar' plan... it's a 'control sugar' plan. It's a way to clean out the artificial level of sweetness you've been tricked into living with, so that you can once again enjoy the natural level of sweetness found in real food.

It's a recalibration of your palate back to what Mother Nature intended, and along the way you can return to a more natural level of healthiness and well being. You'll also increase your odds of eating quite a few more birthday cakes!

So, go forth and enjoy living. Stay alert for hidden and artificial sugars and avoid them like the plague that they've become. Plan your eating to accommodate those wedding cakes... and those s'mores around the campfire... and savor every minute of your sweet success!

Sarah Givens

Made in the USA
Middletown, DE
23 May 2017